Copyright © Stephanie Baker

All rights reserved. No part of this book may be reproduced, scanned or distributed in any printed or electronic form without permission. Please do not participate in or encourage piracy of copyrighted materials in violation of the author's rights. Purchase only authorized editions.

1
EASY RECIPE BROCOLI SOUP

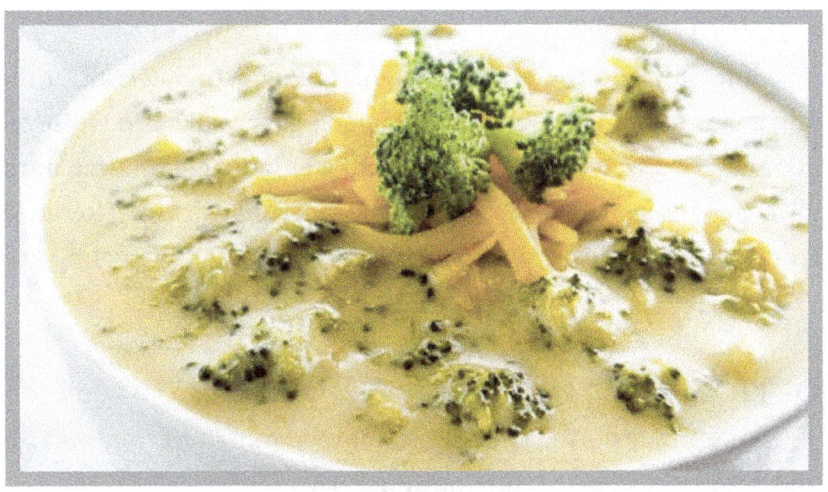

20 MINUTES
   Servings 8

INGREDIENTS

4 cups of broccoli (cut into florets)

4 cloves of garlic (finely chopped)

3 and ha cups chicken stock (or vegetable stock or bone stock)

1 cup of whipped cream

3 cups cheddar cheese (previously grated - see notes)

PREPARATION

Sauté the garlic in a large saucepan over medium heat for one minute until fragrant.

Add the chicken stock, whipped cream and chopped broccoli. Bring heat to a boil, reduce heat and simmer for 10-20 minutes until broccoli is tender.

OPTION 1 (ORIGINAL RECIPE):

Gradually add the grated cheddar cheese, stirring constantly, stirring until melted. (Add half a cup (64 g), simmer and stir until completely dissolved, then repeat half a cup (64 g) at a time until all cheese is gone.) Over high heat to avoid sticking. Remove from heat immediately when all cheese has melted.

OPTION 2 (RECOMMENDED):

make Use a slotted spoon to remove about 1/3 of the broccoli and set aside. (This step is optional if you want to add the last few pieces of soup to the soup. If you want to mix all of the soup, you can leave it there).

USE HAND BLENDER TO blend the remaining broccoli.

. . .

Keep fire to a minimum. attach 1/2 cup of shredded cheddar cheese at a time, stirring constantly, stirring until melted. Mix again to smooth it out.

Remove the stove. Add the broccoli florets reserved for the soup.

2
KETO TURKEY LOW-CARB CHILLI WITHOUT BEANS

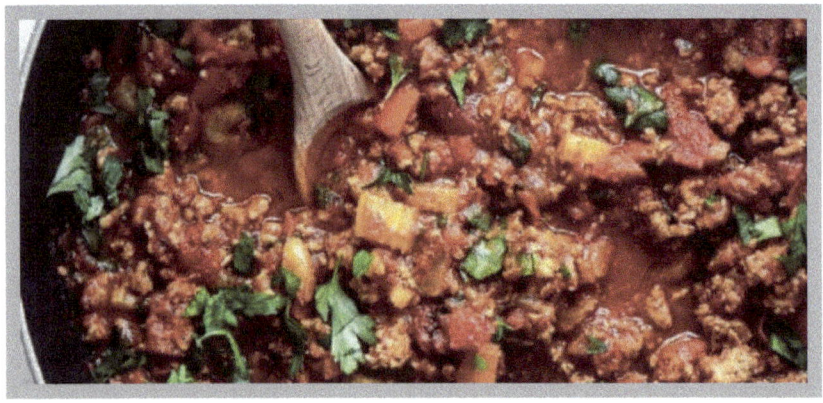

50 MINUTES

INGREDIENTS
1 1/2 tablespoons of olive oil, divided
1/2 cup onion, chopped
1 large red pepper, diced

1/2 cup celery, thinly sliced

1 tablespoon of chopped fresh garlic

1.25 lbs. 93% lean turkey

4 teaspoons of chili powder

1 tablespoon of paprika

1 ½ teaspoon ground cumin

1/4 teaspoon cayenne pepper

1 can of toasted diced tomatoes (14.5 ounces)

1 can of shredded tomatoes (14.5 ounces)

1/2 cup of water

2 tablespoons of tomato paste

1 teaspoon of salt

A pinch of pepper

2 bay leaves

1/4 cup chopped parsley

PREPARATION

In a wide saucepan, heat 1 tablespoon of oil over medium heat. Cook for 3 minutes, or until the onion, bell pepper, celery, and garlic are tender.

Add the rest of the oil and turkey to the pan. Cook until the turkey begins to brown, about 3-4 minutes. Drain the liquid.

Add the spices and cook until the turkey is no longer pink and the spices are fragrant, about 3 to 4 minutes.

Add the fried tomatoes, the chopped tomatoes, the water, the tomato paste, the salt and the pepper and stir until smooth. Then bring to a boil.

After cooking, add the bay leaves, turn the heat on medium and cover the pan. and start Cooking for 30 minutes on low heat, stirring periodically.

Start by removing the bay leaves and add the parsley after the dish has finished cooking.

NUTRITIONAL INFORMATION:

Calories: 195.6 kcal (10%) Carbohydrates: 7.1 g (2%) Protein: 20.6 g (41%) Fat: 10.1 g (16%) Saturated fat: 2.6 g (16%))) Polyunsaturated fat: 0.3 g Monounsaturated fat: 2.5 g Cholesterol: 66 mg (22%) Sodium: 670 mg (29%) Potassium: 222.1 mg (6%) Dietary fiber: 2 g (8 %)) Sugar: 3 g (3%) Vitamin A: 27.1 IU (1%) Vitamin C: 73.1 mg (89%) Calcium: 2.2 mg Iron: 4 mg (22%)

③
CHICKEN AND AVOCADO SOUP

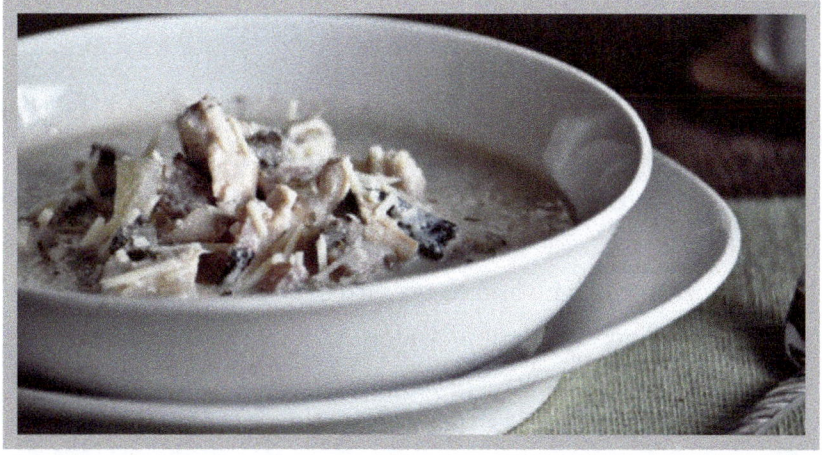

25 min

servings 4

INGREDIENTS

2 teaspoons olive oil

1-1/2 cups finely chopped shallots
2 garlic cloves, minced
1 medium tomato, diced
5 cups reduced sodium chicken broth
2 cups shredded chicken breast, 12 ounces
8 ounces of 2 small ripe avocados, diced
1/3 cup cilantro, chopped
4 lime wedges
kosher salt and fresh pepper, just enough
1/8 teaspoon cumin
Pinch of chipotle chili powder, optional

PREPARATION

Heat a large saucepan over medium heat.

Add the oil, 1 cup of the shallots, and the garlic. Fry for 2 to 3 minutes until tender, then add the tomatoes and cook for another minute until tender.

Add the chicken broth, cumin, and chili powder and bring to a boil. Cook over low heat for about 15 minutes.

Put 1/2 cup of the chicken, 1/2 avocado, the rest of the shallot and the cilantro in each of the four bowls. Pour 1 cup of chicken broth over the chicken and serve with a lemon wedge.

Serving Size: 13/4 cups, Calories: 297kcal, Carbohydrates: 14.5g, Protein: 31g, Fat: 14g, Saturated Fat: 2.5g, Cholesterol: 72.5mg, Sodium: 789.5mg, Fiber: 7.5g , sugar: 2.5g Blue Smart Points: 4 Green Smart Points: 6 Purple Smart Points: 4 + Points: 7

4
SHRIMP AND BACON SOUP

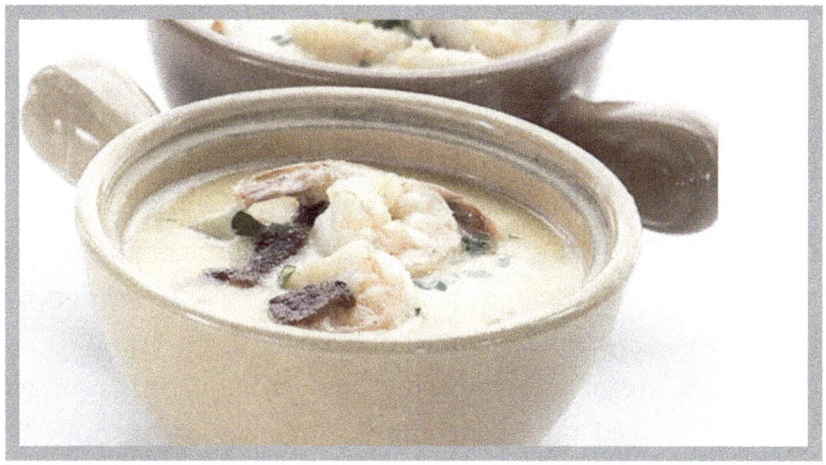

30 MINUTES
Servings 6

INGREDIENTS

6 slices of bacon, chopped
1 medium turnip cut into 1/2 inch cubes
½ cup onion, chopped
2 cloves of garlic, minced
2 cups of chicken broth
1 cup heavy whipping cream
1 pound peeled and cleaned shrimp, with or without a tail
½ teaspoon of cajun seasoning
salt and pepper
Chopped parsley for garnish

PREPARATION

IN A BIGSAUCEPAN OR DUTCH OVEN, cook the bacon over medium heat until crisp. Deplete on a paper towel-lined plate with a slotted spoon and keep the bacon fat in the pan.

In a large skillet, sauté the beets and onion for about 5 minutes, or until the onion is tender. Cook for about a minute, or until the garlic becomes fragrant. Cook, stirring occasionally, till the beets are tender, about 10 minutes.

Add the cream and prawns and simmer until the prawns are pink and cooked through, another 3 minutes or so. Add the Cajun seasoning and season with salt and pepper.

Garnish with bacon and chopped parsley after serving.

Remarks

Tip: Some Cajun spices contain a lot of salt. After adding the seasonings, taste the soup before adding more salt and pepper. Also, make sure the dressing doesn't contain sugar or other fillers. We really like Slap Ya Mama Spice Mix. Yes, that's what it really says!

nutrition

Serving size: 1 serving = about 3/4 cup | Calories: 391 kcal | Carbohydrates: 5.6 g | Protein: 16.5 g | Fat: 31.9 g | Fiber: 0.6 g

5
KETO BEEF STEW

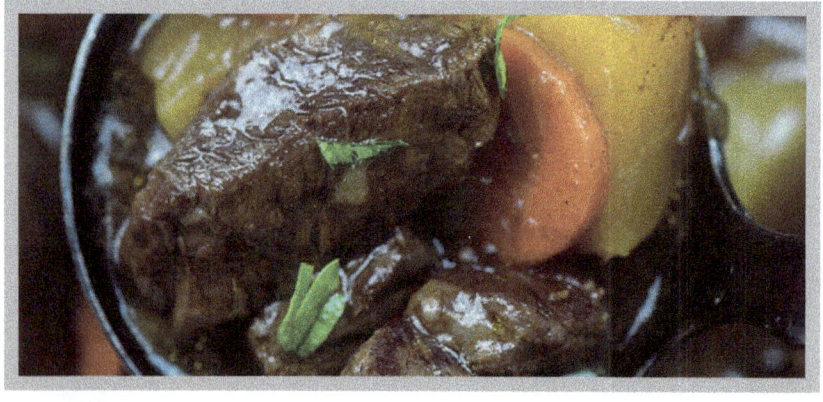

2 HOURS and 50 minutes
Servings 6

INGREDIENTS
1 ½ pounds of roasted chuck, diced
1 tablespoon avocado oil, more if needed

3 teaspoons of salt, divided

4 1/2 cups beef broth, divided

2 tablespoons of red wine vinegar

2 tablespoons of tomato paste

1 tablespoon of Worcestershire sauce

1 large bay leaf

1 pound beetroot, peeled and chopped

2 medium carrots, peeled and cut into coins

1 medium onion, diced

1 stick of celery, chopped

2 cloves of garlic, minced

½ teaspoon of xanthan gum

1 tablespoon of chopped fresh parsley

PREPARATION

Preheat a large Dutch oven over medium-high heat. Add the oil and heat until bright.

Sprinkle the meat with 1 teaspoon of salt. Add the meat to the pot in a single layer (you will likely need to work in batches) and cook for about 5 minutes per batch until golden brown on all sides. Add more oil between batches as needed. Put all the meat in a bowl and set aside.

Place half a cup of the beef stock and vinegar in the Dutch oven and scrape the golden pieces into the bottom of the pan over medium-high heat.

Return the meat to the pan with the beef stock, tomato paste, Worcestershire sauce, and bay leaf. Bring to a boil, bring to a boil and cover. Cook over low heat for 1 1/2 hours or until the meat is tender.

Add the beets, carrots, onions, celery, garlic and the

remaining 2 teaspoons of salt. Stir to combine.

Take half a cup of liquid from the saucepan into a small bowl or measuring cup. Sprinkle with xanthan gum and beat well. Return the mixture to the saucepan and simmer, uncovered, for 45 minutes or until vegetables are tender, stirring occasionally.

Remove the bay leaf and sprinkle with parsley before serving.
Remarks

Smaller beets tend to be sweeter than larger beets and have a less bitter taste.

You can use half a glass of dry red wine instead of beef broth to degrease the pan.

I have not measured the portions by volume. Distribute evenly in six bowls.

6
EASY KETO FRENCH ONION SOUP (RICH AND CHEESY)

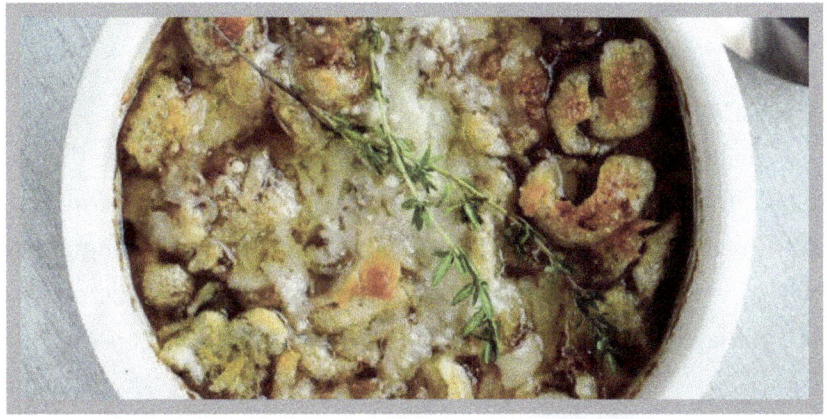

45 MINUTES

INGREDIENTS
¾ cup of salted butter

½ cup of slicedyellow onions
¼ cup of green onions, chopped
1 teaspoon of erythritol or 2-4 drops of liquid stevia
2 cloves of garlic, chopped
1/8 teaspoon of xanthan gum
4 cups of beef stock
1 tablespoon of apple cider vinegar
1 or 2 sprigs of fresh thyme
1 bay leaf
½ teaspoon of fine sea salt
¼ teaspoon ground black pepper
200 g bark
½ cup of Gruyere cheese, chopped
½ cup of grated Parmesan cheese

PREPARATION

Inside a medium saucepan use medium heat, melt the butter. Cook for 8-10 minutes, until the yellow and green onions are translucent. Add the erythritol and cook, stirring frequently with a wooden spoon, for around 5 minutes, or until the onions are golden brown.

ADD the garlic and xanthan gum and mix well, then add the stock, vinegar, thyme, bay leaf, salt and pepper. Cover and simmer for about 20 minutes.

MEANWHILE, preheat the grill. Cut each shell into 3-4 "croutons."

. . .

DIVIDE THE STOCK into 4 cups. Cover each bowl with a quarter of the crust and 2 tablespoons of each cheese. Grill until cheese has melted.

7
KETO STROGANOFF SOUP

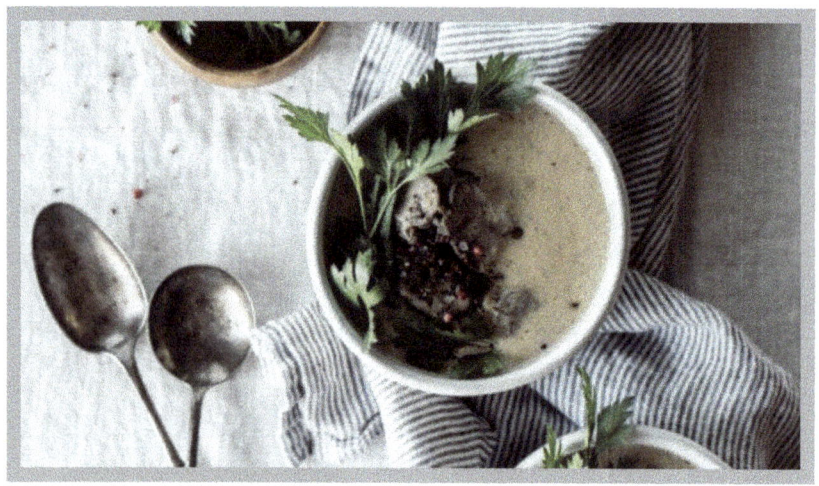

6 HOURS and 30 minutes
Servings 12

INGREDIENTS

4 cups of beef broth

10 ounces of cremini mushrooms, thinly sliced

1 medium onion, diced

4 minced garlic cloves

3 tablespoons of butter

1 teaspoon of sea salt

1 ½ pound sirloin steak, thinly sliced (get my grass-fed beef here)

1 cup of whipped cream

1 cup of sour cream

2 tablespoons of beef broth

2 tablespoons of Dijon mustard

2 tablespoons of fresh parsley, finely chopped

1 ½ teaspoon of onion powder (I use this brand of herbs)

1 ½ teaspoon of garlic powder

1 teaspoon of dried oregano

PREPARATION

Heat the slow cooker over high heat. Place the beef stock and mushrooms in the slow cooker and cover.

Heat the butter in a large skillet over medium heat. put the onion and garlic to the pan and sauté until the onion turns translucent and the garlic is fragrant. Add them to the slow cooker.

Sprinkle the sirloin with salt, add it to the pan and brown on both sides for about 2 minutes.

PLACE THE STEAK, whipped cream, sour cream, beef broth, Dijon, parsley, onion powder, garlic powder, and oregano into the slow cooker. Cover and cook over high heat for 6 hours.

DEGREES

Visit my friends at the Butcher Box for delicious grass-fed, grass-ready beef, organic chicken, and free range pork. Jon and I have been eating Butcher Box meat for over 2 years and it is the best meat we have ever eaten.

NUTRITION

Serving Size: 1 cup Calories: 300 Fat: 19g Carbohydrates: 4.5g Net Protein: 20g

8
CHICKEN SOUP WITH ZUCCHINI NOODLES

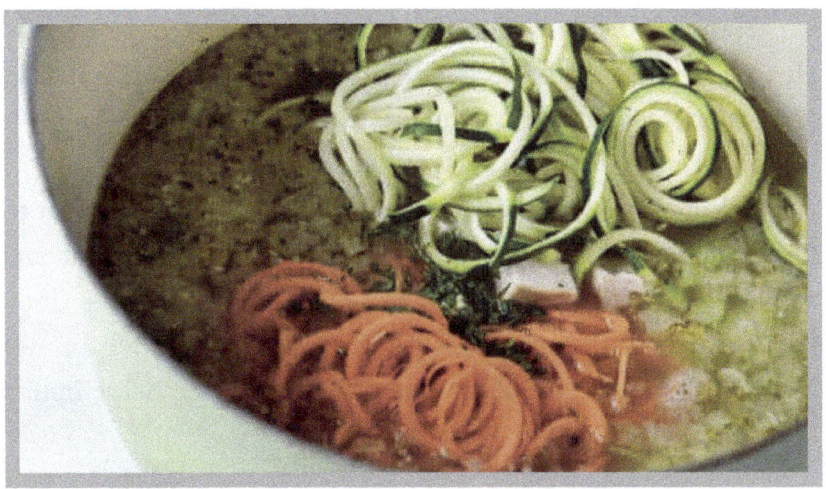

40 MINUTES
Servings 2

INGREDIENTS

2 tablespoons of olive oil

1 1/2 large garlic cloves, minced

2 celery stalks, halved lengthwise and finely chopped

1/2 medium white onion, chopped

4 cups of low sodium chicken broth

4 sprigs of thyme

1/2 teaspoon of dried oregano

1 teaspoon of chopped fresh parsley

2 cups of chicken cutlet on the baking sheet

1 large carrot, peeled and rolled

1 large courgette, twisted

PREPARATION

Heat olive oil in a large saucepan medium heat. When the oil glistens, add the garlic, celery and onion. Season with salt and pepper and cook for 3-5 minutes, stirring or until the onion is transparent and the vegetables soften.

Add the broth, thyme, oregano and parsley. Raise the heat to high and bring the soup to a boil, then bring to a boil and simmer for 5 minutes. Add the chicken and carrot noodles. Cook for 5 minutes, then put the zucchini noodles and cook for another 1 to 2 minutes until all noodles are tender. Serve immediately.

9
CREAMY SOUP WITH CHICKEN AND BROCCOLI

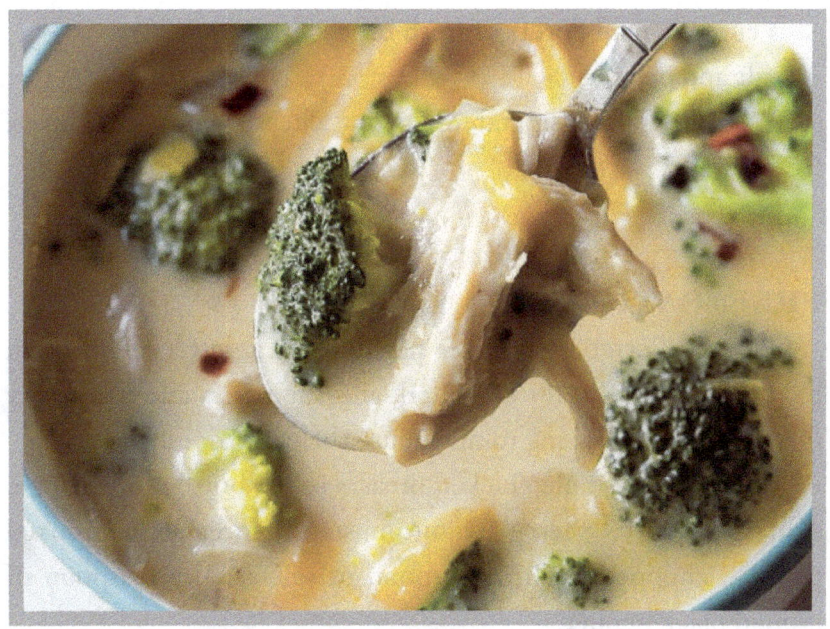

35 MINUTES
Servings 6

. . .

INGREDIENTS

1 large onion, finely chopped
3 minced garlic cloves
1 tablespoon of butter
1 pound of boneless chicken breast
8 cups of low sodium chicken broth
3 tablespoons of dry sherry
2 tablespoons of Dijon mustard
1 teaspoon of cornstarch
1/2 teaspoon of smoked paprika
1/4 tsp ground red pepper
4 ounces of low-fat cream cheese, diced
3 cups of small florets of fresh broccoli
salt and pepper

Possible toppings: grated low-fat cheese, chopped chives, fresh parsley

PREPARATION

Put the butter in a 4-liter pot and let it rest over medium heat. When the butter is melted, add the onion and garlic. Fry for 3-4 minutes, stirring to make sure the garlic doesn't burn.

position the whole chicken breasts in the bottom of the pan. Add the broth, sherry, Dijon mustard, cornstarch, smoked paprika, chopped chilli, 1 teaspoon of salt and 1/2 teaspoon of ground black pepper.

Bring the broth to a boil. Reduce the heat, cover and simmer for 15-20 minutes to cook the chicken.

Remove the chicken breast with the tongs. Then add the

cream cheese. Whisk to melt the cream cheese in the broth. Then use two forks to chop the chicken.

Add the broccoli florets and grated chicken to the soup. Stir well and turn off the heat. The broccoli florets cook quickly in the hot broth.

Season to taste and season with salt and pepper. Serve hot.

10

KALE SOUP WITH SLOW COOKER SAUSAGE

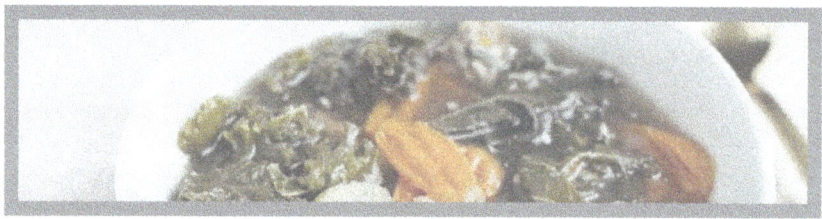

6 HOURS 15 minutes
servings 4

INGREDIENTS

3 cloves of garlic, chopped
1 large onion, finely chopped
2 cups of carrots, chopped
2 celery stalks, chopped
2 32-ounce boxes of chicken stock or stock (about 8 cups)
1 teaspoon of pepper

1/4 teaspoon salt or more to taste
4 cups of cabbage, chopped
1 pound sage sausage
Parmesan cheese to serve (optional)

PREPARATION

Cook the sausage in a large skillet or saucepan over medium heat while breaking it into pieces. Start by removing them with a slotted spoon when golden brown and drain on a plate lined with absorbent material. Remove all but 1 tablespoon of the fat from the pan.

IN THE RESERVED FAT, cook garlic, onion, carrots, and celery for 4-5 minutes, or until fragrant.

In a slow cooker, combine the vegetables, stock, pepper, and salt, and mix in the sausage.

Continue cooking for 3 hours on high or 6 hours on low. Put the kale in the slow cooker 10 minutes before serving.

Season with more salt, pepper, and Parmesan cheese and serve in bowls.

NUTRITION
Serving Size: 1/4 of the recipe
Calories: 479 |
Sugar: 7 g |
Fat: 31 g |
Carbohydrates: 12 g |
Fiber: 3g |
Protein: 34 g

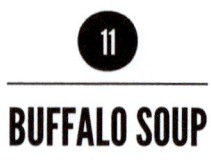

BUFFALO SOUP

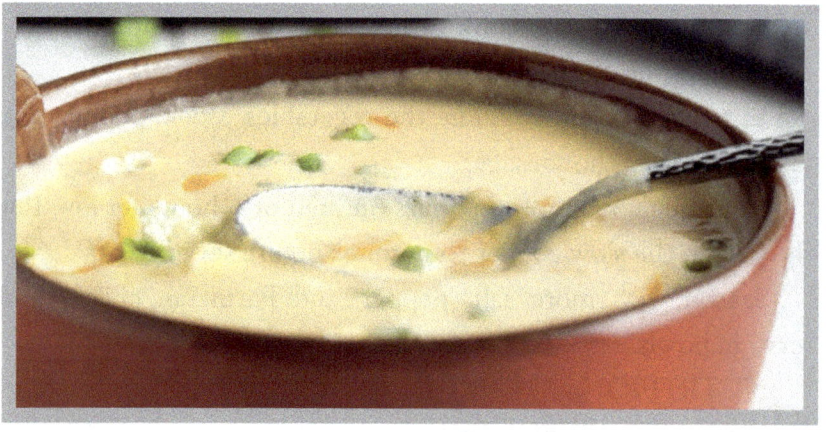

45 MINUTES
Servings: 12

INGREDIENTS

1 tablespoon of oil or butter
1 big sweet onion, peeled and finely chopped
4 cloves of garlic, peeled and finely chopped
6 cups of cauliflower florets
5 cups of vegetable stock
1/4 cup hot buffalo sauce (such as Frank's RedHot)
6 ounces of cream cheese
1 cup of cheddar cheese shredded
salt and pepper

Possible toppings: extra cheese, blue cheese, pieces of bacon, chives

PREPARATION

Place a large 6-liter saucepan over medium heat. Add the oil, chopped onion and garlic. Brown for 3 minutes. Then add the cauliflower and fry for another 5-7 minutes, stirring occasionally so that the garlic doesn't burn.

POUR the vegetable stock and buffalo sauce into the pan. Cover the soup and simmer for at least 20 minutes, or until the largest cauliflower flowers are tender.

Carefully pour the hot soup into a blender. Add the cream cheese and grated cheddar cheese. Place the lid on the blender and open the opening on the lid. Place a tea towel in the mixer to let the steam escape. However, do not splash hot soup through the open opening. Then mix until you get a homogeneous mixture.

and Taste it and season with salt and pepper if necessary.

Serve warm, sprinkled with extra cheese, spring onions (or bacon if you eat meat)!

Serving Size: 1 Cup, Calories: 104 kcal, Carbs: 7g, Protein: 4g, Fat: 6g, Saturated Fat: 3g, Cholesterol: 17mg, Sodium: 687mg, Potassium: 230mg, Fiber: 1g , Sugar: 4g, Vitamin A: 380IU, Vitamin C: 25.7mg, Calcium: 107mg, Iron: 0.4mg

12

CREAMY LOW-CARB CHICKEN AND MUSHROOM SOUP

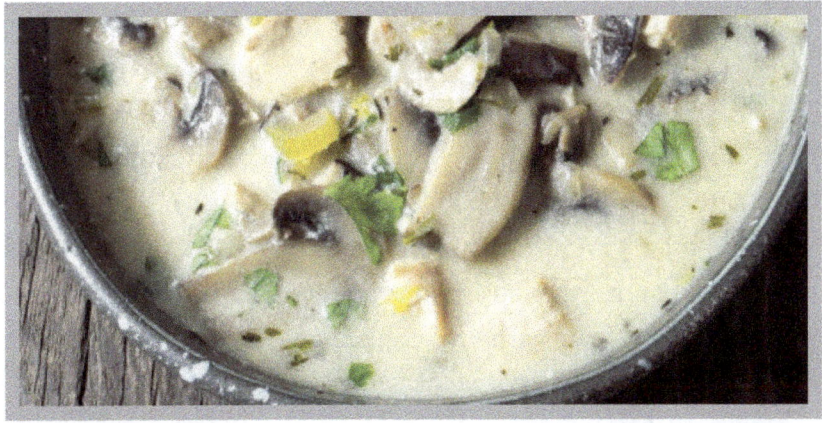

33 MINUTES
Servings: 8

INGREDIENTS

2 tablespoons of unsalted butter
1 lbig sweet onion, peeled and finely chopped
1 cup of chopped celery
5-6 cloves of garlic, peeled and finely chopped
18 grams of sliced mushrooms, mixed varieties
1 teaspoon of chopped fresh rosemary
1 teaspoon of dried thyme
1/3 cup of dry sherry
1 pound boneless chicken breast
8 cups of chicken stock
2/3 cup of whipped cream
1 tablespoon cornstarch (or arrowroot for keto)
1/4 cup of chopped parsley
salt and pepper

PREPARATION

PUT the butter in a large 6-8 liter pan and heat over medium heat. After melting, add the onions, celery and garlic.

Saute for 2-3 minutes then add the mushrooms, rosemary and thyme. Sauté until the mushrooms are tender and cook.

Deglaze the pan with the dry sherry. Then add the whole chicken breast, chicken stock, 1 teaspoon of salt and 1/4 teaspoon of black pepper. Bring to the boil. Then reduce the heat and simmer for 15 minutes or until the chicken fillet is cooked.

When the chicken is cooked, use the tongs to remove the breast and cut it into small pieces.

Add the cornstarch to the cream taking care not to form lumps. Then beat the cream in the pan and let it simmer and thicken. Add the chicken mince to the soup and add the parsley. Then taste salt and pepper if necessary.

Serving Size: 1.5 Cups, Calories: 215kcal, Carbohydrates: 9g, Protein: 16g, Fat: 12g, Saturated Fat: 6g, Cholesterol: 70mg, Sodium: 952mg, Potassium: 722mg, Fiber: 1 g, sugar: 3 g, vitamin A: 610 IU, vitamin C: 24 mg, calcium: 53 mg, iron: 1.5 mg

13
CIOPPINO SEAFOOD RECIPE

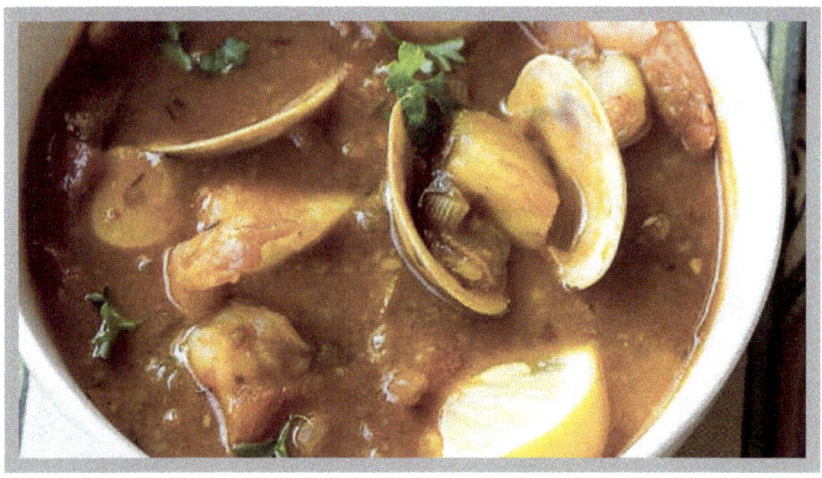

1 HOUR 5 minutes
Servings: 8

INGREDIENTS

2 tablespoons of olive oil
1 large fennel, thinly sliced
1 large onion, chopped
6 cloves of garlic, sliced
3 tablespoons of tomato paste
1 tablespoon of dried tarragon or 2 tablespoons of fresh tarragon
4-5 sprigs of fresh thyme
1 large pinch of saffron
1/2 teaspoon of ground red pepper
1 bay leaf
2 teaspoons of salt
1 1/2 cups of wine (fruity red or dry white)
28 grams of diced tomatoes
32 grams of sea broth
1 1/2 pounds of scallops or scallops

1 POUND hard-boiled white fish
1 pound of raw peeled shrimp
1-2 tablespoons of flour
Lemon wedges and chopped parsley for garnish

PREPARATION

Prepare the fennel: cut the stems. You can use the sheets later in the week. (Think of salads, sauces, mixed with goat cheese, sprinkled with fruit ...) Then cut the onion in half and core. Cut the light bulb into thin slices. With smaller panes, you can divide the lightbulb into quarters.

Put a large saucepan over medium heat. Add 2 tablespoons of

oil to the pan. Fry the fennel and onion for 5 minutes; Then add the garlic and tomato paste.

Suffer another minute. And season to taste with tarragon, thyme, saffron, chili, bay leaf, salt, and black pepper. Mix thoroughly. Pour the wine, broth, and tomatoes into the pot. Toss the stew in a pot with enough water to cover it and bring to a boil. Reduce the heat to minimum, cover, and cook for 30 minutes.

In the meantime, cut the fish into 1 inch cubes and mix the flour with the fish and prawns. Rinse and check all shellfish to see if they are fresh. Everything has to be completely closed. When they are open, tighten them. If they don't close immediately, throw them away. Open or cracked molluscs must not get into the Cioppino.

When the stew has cooked for more than 30 minutes, add the shellfish. Stir and cook for 3-5 minutes until almost open. Then add the fish and prawns. Stir well and simmer for another 3-5 minutes. The broth should be thickened and all shellfish should be wide open.

Start by removing the thyme sprigs, bay leaf, and any shellfish that haven't been opened. Serve the cioppino with lemon wedges and parsley on top. And serve with sourdough bread or Parmesan toast that is soft and crispy.

CALORIES: 258 kcal, carbohydrates: 13 g, protein: 29 g, fat: 6 g, saturated fat: 1 g, cholesterol: 175 mg, sodium: 1696 mg, potassium: 784 mg, fiber: 3 g, sugar: 4 g , Vitamin A: 375 IU, Vitamin C.: 19.2 mg, Calcium: 197 mg, Iron: 4 mg

14

PALEO GREEN CHILI CHICKEN

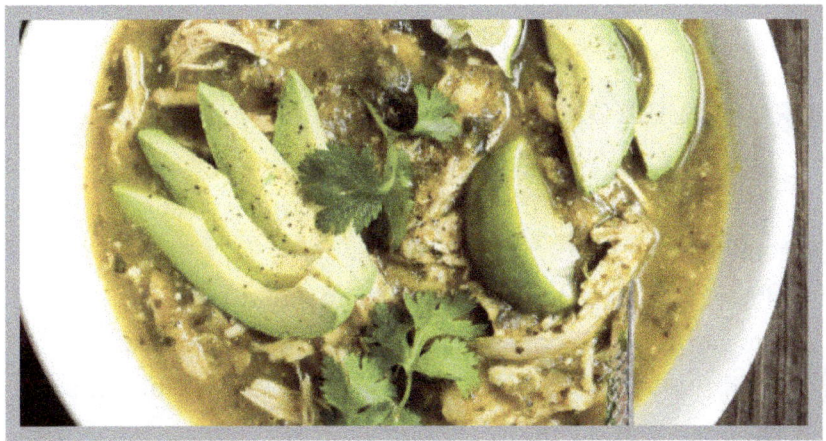

1 HOUR

Servings: 8

INGREDIENTS

2 tablespoons olive oil

1 large onion, peeled and minced

6 garlic cloves, peeled and minced

4 poblano peppers, seeded and minced

1-2 jalapeno peppers, seeded and minced

1 pound of tomatoes

1 tablespoon ground cumin

1 tablespoon ground coriander

1 tablespoon dried oregano

1 teaspoon salt

1 bay leaf

2 1/2 pounds boneless chicken (breast, thighs, or both)

4 cups of chicken broth

1/2 cup coriander chopped

Possible garnishes: coriander, avocado, lime.

PREPARATION

Peel and wash the tomatoes so they don't get sticky. Then cut the tomatoes into quarters. Prepare the remaining vegetables.

Put a large 6-liter saucepan over medium heat. Add the oil, onion, garlic, and chopped peppers. Fry for 5-8 minutes.

Add the tomatoes. Next, place the whole raw chicken pieces in the pot. Add all the seasonings and seasonings. Pour in the broth. Stir and slide the chicken pieces to the bottom of the pot.

Boil the chili for 25-30 minutes, until the largest piece of chicken is cooked through. Use the tongs to move the chicken pieces on a cutting board.

Remove the bay leaf. Then use an immersion blender to blend the vegetables and broth.Everything doesn't have to be absolutely smooth, but the tomato chunks should be mixed in.

Meanwhile, shred the chicken with two forks. After that, toss the chicken cutlet with the chili.

Taste it, then season with salt and pepper as needed. Finally, add the chopped cilantro. Serve hot as is or with lemon wedges and sliced avocado.

Observations

Don't have a hand mixer yet?

Use a large slotted spoon to scoop tomatoes, onions, and bell peppers into a standard blender. For safety reasons, open the ventilation grill and the lid with a towel. Mashed potatoes. Then mix the vegetable mixture with the broth.

⬤15

10 MINUTE TOMATO BASIL SOUP

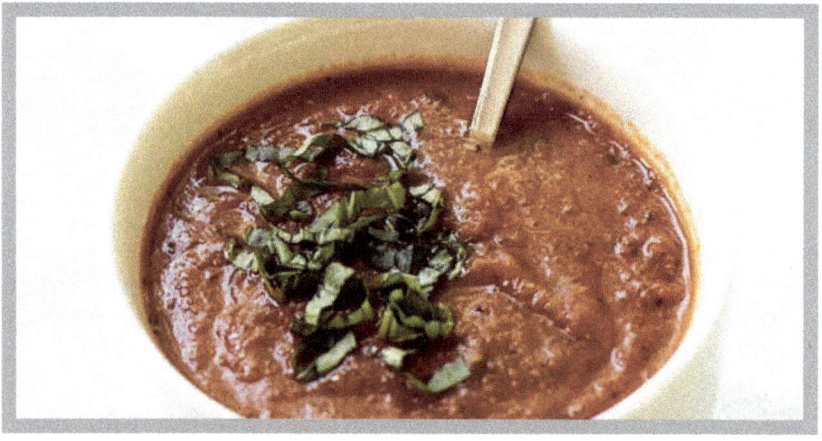

Yield in 10 minutes
  Serving 1

INGREDIENTS
  2 teaspoons olive oil

1 teaspoon minced garlic
1/4 cup onion, minced
1 (14.5 oz) can cook roasted tomato cubes (see note)
1/3 cup chicken broth
2 large basil leaves, chopped
Salt to taste

PREPARATION

Heat olive oil in a saucepan and use medium heat. Add garlic and onion and cook for a minute or until garlic becomes fragrant. Add the tomatoes and the broth. Let the soup simmer for five minutes.

Blend the soup with a hand mixer or put it in a planetary mixer. Add the basil, mix, season with salt and serve.

OBSERVATIONS

In this recipe, the kind of canned tomatoes you use makes a huge difference. Since Muir Glen tomatoes are sweeter and less acidic, I like them.

KETO BACON SHRIMP SOUP

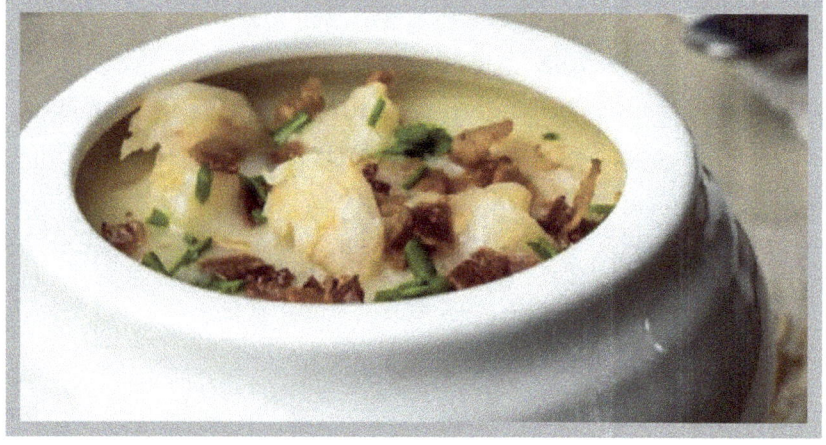

25 MINUTES

Sevings 6

INGREDIENTS

1 pound peeled and peeled shrimp (chopped)

1/2 pound of bacon

3 cups of chicken broth

1 1/2 cups heavy whipping cream

1/4 cup finely chopped onion

2 teaspoons of freshly ground black pepper

2 teaspoons of smoked paprika

pink Himalayan salt

PREPARATION

In a big skillet, cook the bacon until crisp.

Remove the bacon and crumble it after it has cooled.

Add the onion to the pan with the bacon fat and gently sauté it.

Combine the chicken stock, whipped cream, salt, pepper, and paprika in a large mixing bowl.

Take the mixture to a boil, stirring constantly, until it thickens.

Toss in the shrimp and bacon crumbles.

Cook until the shrimp are pink and the soup has reached the perfect consistency over low heat.

Serve in a bowl and warm the bones!

17
EASY BURGER STEW WITH SLOW COOKER OPTION

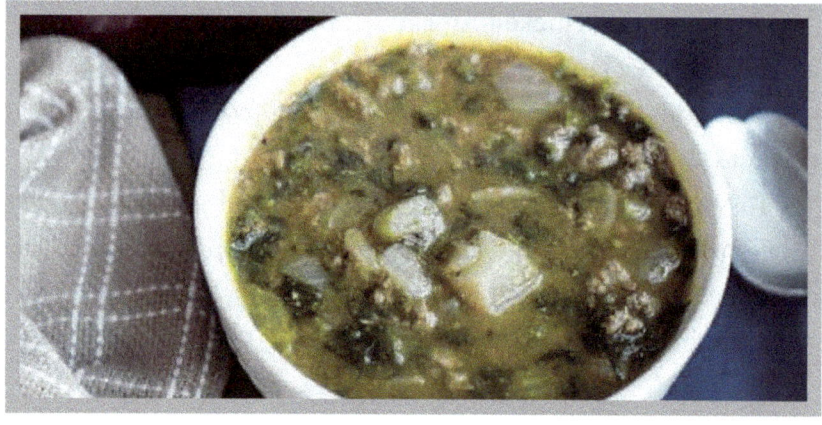

1 HOUR
   Servings 10

INGREDIENTS
   2 tablespoons of olive oil

2 pounds of grass-fed ground beef or venison

1 small onion, chopped

3 cloves of garlic, minced

32 grams of beef broth

15 ounces of canned or fresh pumpkin puree

10 grams of radishes, chopped

4 celery sticks, sliced

1 ½ tablespoon of sea salt

Skip 1 teaspoon of ground black pepper for AIP

1 teaspoon of dried oregano

1 teaspoon of dried basil

1 teaspoon of parsley flakes

½ teaspoon of marjoram

¼ teaspoon of sage

10 grams of chopped spinach (fresh or frozen)

PREPARATION

Working hours:

In a pan, heat oil by applying medium heat. Combine the minced beef, onion, and garlic in a mixing bowl. Cook until the meat has become golden brown.

Add the broth, pumpkin, radish, celery and herbs. Bring to the boil. Lower the heat and simmer, covered, for 20 minutes.

Add the spinach and cook, covered, for another 10 minutes. Adjust the covers as needed.

Stew:

Fry the ground beef with onion and garlic and add it to the slow cooker if needed.

Combine the broth, pumpkin, radish, celery, and herbs in a

large mixing bowl. Cook for 4-6 hours on low heat. Apply the spinach in the last 1-2 hours of cooking.

Bachelor's degree

In lieu of spinach, cabbage or kale may be used. Radishes may be attached to cabbage. After the cabbage leaves and spinach have been cooked, they are added.

Low Carb Sweeteners | Ketogenic Sweetener Conversion Table

5 LOW CARB ingredients in Yum Keto

nutrition

Serving size: 1 cup | Calories: 301 | Carbohydrates: 7 g | Protein: 20 g | Fat: 21 g | Saturated fat: 7 g | Cholesterol: 64 mg | Sodium: 1190 mg | Potassium: 612 mg | Fiber: 2 g | Sugar: 2 g | Vitamin A: 9350 IU | Vitamin C: 15.3 mg | Calcium: 78 mg | Iron: 3.4 mg

WHOLE CABBAGE SOUP 30

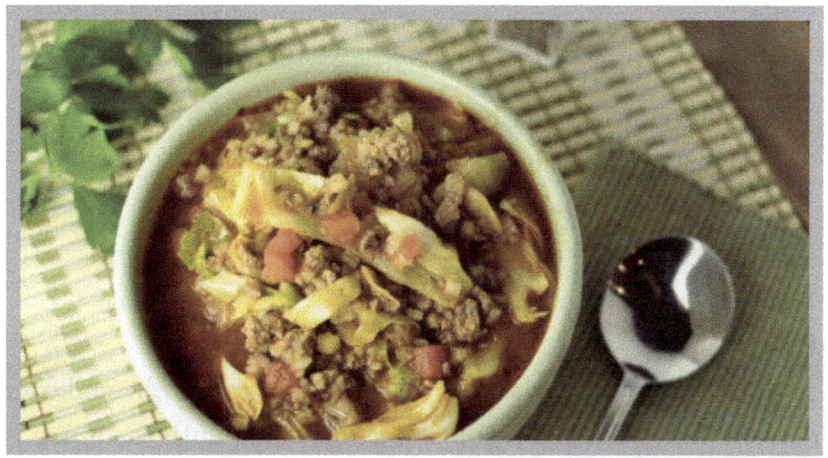

1 HOUR

Serving 6

INGREDIENTS

2 tablespoons of butter or ghee (I use this brand of ghee)
2 tablespoons of olive oil
1 cup onion, chopped
4 cloves of garlic, minced
1 ½ pounds of ground beef (get my grass-fed beef here)
½ pound of ground pork
6 cups of beef broth
3 teaspoons of dried oregano leaves (I use this brand)
2 teaspoons of sea salt
2 teaspoons of smoked paprika
2 teaspoons of garlic powder
2 teaspoons of onion powder
1 teaspoon of black pepper
½ tsp dried thyme (I use this brand)
(2) 14.5-ounce cans of diced tomatoes, drained
6 ounces of tomato paste
2 tablespoons of chopped fresh parsley
1 large cabbage, halved and sliced
3 cups of cauliflower with rice

PREPARATION

In a large skillet or skillet, heat the butter and olive oil over medium heat. Add the onion and garlic. Cook until the onion is translucent and the garlic is fragrant.

Add the ground beef and pork to the pan. Cook until golden brown and excess fat to drain. Add the meat stock, oregano, sea salt, paprika, garlic powder, onion powder, black pepper, thyme, tomatoes, tomato paste, parsley, cabbage and cauliflower with rice. Put to the, boil then turn down to a low heat and cook for another 30-45 minutes.

DEGREE

6.5g net carbs per serving

NUTRITION

Serving Size: 1 cup Calories: 200 Fat: 12.9g Carbs: 10.5g Net Fiber: 4g Protein: 12.1g

19

KETO CHICKEN CORDON BLEU SOUP

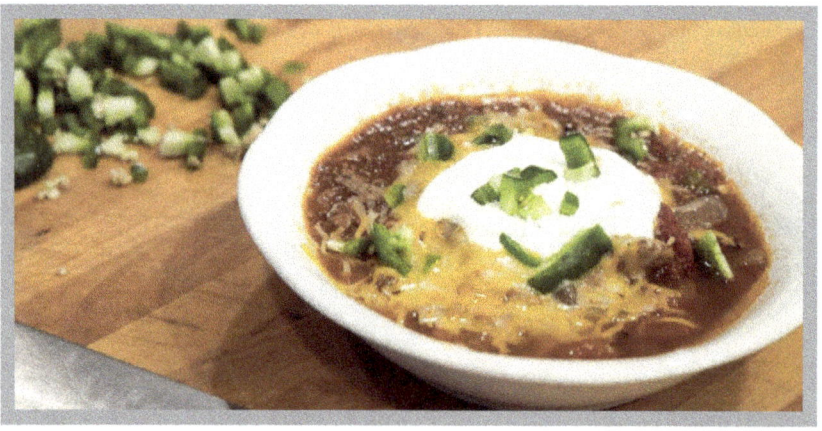

6 hours and 30 minutes.
Servings 16

INGREDIENTS
6 cups of chicken broth

12 ounces diced ham
5 ounces mushrooms, chopped
4 ounces onion, diced
2 teaspoons dried tarragon
1 teaspoon sea salt, more to taste
1 teaspoon black pepper
1 pound chicken breast, diced
4 garlic cloves, minced
3 tablespoons salted butter
1 ½ cup heavy cream
½ cup sour cream
½ cup grated Parmesan cheese
4 ounces Swiss cheese

PREPARATION

Heat the slow cooker to a low setting.

In the slow cooker, add the chicken broth, ham, mushrooms, onion, tarragon, salt, and pepper. Cover and cook.

In a large skillet over medium heat, fry the chicken in butter and garlic until golden. Place the chicken in the slow cooker along with the drippings from the skillet.

Then add the cream, sour cream, Parmesan, and Swiss cheese. Cover and simmer for 6 hours.

OBSERVATIONS

Per serving - Calories: 178 | Fat: 12 g | Proteins: 16 g | Net carbs: 2.75 g

NUTRITION

Serving size: 1 cup

20
LOW CARB CHICKEN TACO SOUP

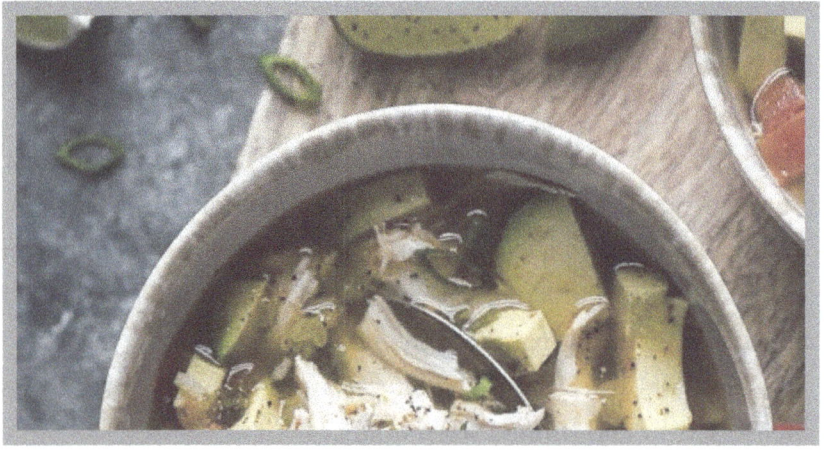

38 MINUTES
Servings 4

INGREDIENTS
1 pound chicken breast

1/2 cup onion, chopped
4 garlic cloves, minced
1 tablespoon of chipotles in adobo sauce, chopped
1 tablespoon of cumin
½ teaspoon chili powder
½ teaspoon of paprika
½ teaspoon of salt
2 tablespoons lemon juice
1 tablespoon lime juice
2 cups of chicken broth
8 ounces cream cheese
½ cup cilantro, chopped

PREPARATION

Instant pot method

Place chicken, onion, garlic, chipotles, cumin, chili powder, paprika, salt, lemon juice, lime juice, and chicken broth in an Instant Pot.

Cover, twist vent to seal, and cook on high pressure for 18 minutes.

allow the pressure release naturally for about 10 minutes before removing the lid.

Remove the chicken from the pot and use two forks to chop it.

Turn the Instant Pot to brown and add the cream cheese. Whisk continuously until cream cheese is completely melted and incorporated.

Turn off the Instant Pot and place the chicken back in the pot. Add the cilantro and mix well to combine.

Serve immediately

Slow cook method

Bring the chicken, onion, garlic, chipotles, cumin, chili powder, paprika, salt, lemon juice, lime juice, and chicken broth over low heat.

Cover and simmer for 4 hours.

Remove the chicken from the pot and use two forks to chop it.

Put the cream cheese in the slow cooker and beat constantly until the cream cheese is completely melted and incorporated.

Return the chicken to the slow cooker and add the cilantro. Stir well to combine.

SERVE IMMEDIATELY.

Observations

This soup is great with shredded cheddar cheese, cilantro, sour cream, and diced tomatoes. However, the nutritional information does not contain spices.

21
CHICKEN NOODLE SOUP

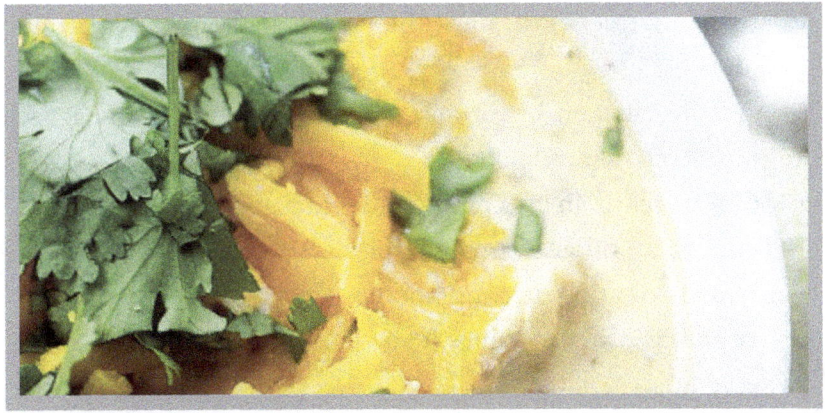

30 MINUTES

Servings 6

INGREDIENTS

2 tablespoons of olive oil

½ sweet onion, chopped

3 stalks of celery cut into cubes

1 diced red pepper

1 finely chopped garlic clove

6 cups of chicken broth

2 cups cooked chicken, shredded

½ teaspoon of dried oregano

½ teaspoon of dried basil

1 teaspoon of salt

1 teaspoon of ground pepper

4 large courgettes

PREPARATION

Start by Heat the olive oil in a big skillet or saucepan over medium heat.

Add the onion, celery, bell pepper, and garlic to the pan and cook, stirring frequently, until the vegetables are tender, around 5 minutes.

Add the chicken broth and chicken to the pan along with oregano, basil, salt and pepper.

Spiral zucchini in zucchini noodles and add them to the pan.

Bring to a boil and simmer. Simmer for 10 minutes, stirring occasionally, or until zucchini noodles are as soft as desired.

Try adding other toppings if you like.

Serve hot.

BEEF SOUP WITH VEGETABLES AND CABBAGE

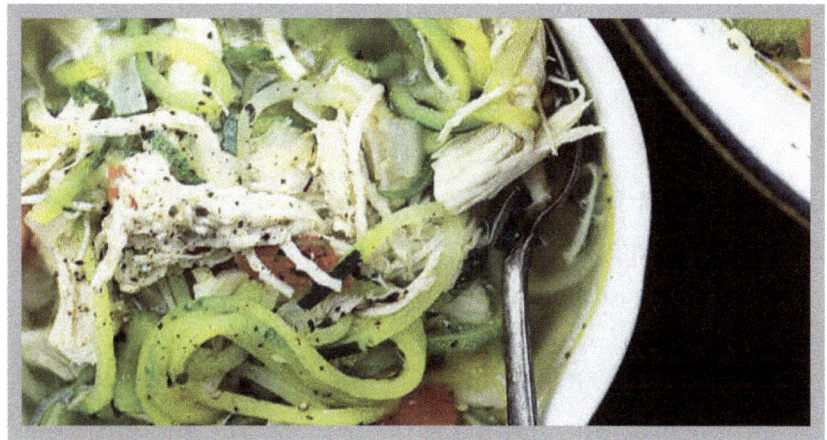

1 HOUR and 25 minutes
Serving 6

INGREDIENTS
1.5 pounds of roast beef

3 tablespoons of olive oil

2 cups of chopped cabbage

1 tablespoon of tomato paste

1 red pepper

1 spring onion

2 cloves of garlic

½ teaspoon of cayenne pepper

1 teaspoon of broth powder

1 teaspoon of thyme

1 teaspoon ground shrimp substitute with 1 tablespoon of coconut amino acids

1 teaspoon of salt to taste

2 cups of beef broth

2 cups of water

A pinch of black pepper to brown the meat.

A pinch of salt to brown the meat.

PREPARATION

Chop the cabbage, chives, garlic and paprika.

Cut the meat into pieces if it is not already cut.

Turn on the Instant Pot and switch to Sauté mode.

Add the olive oil and then the meat.

pa pinch of salt and black pepper and stir the meat until golden brown.

Add the green onions and garlic and mix until tender.

Add the red pepper, tomato puree and all the spices.

Pour in 2 cups of meat broth and 2 cups of water.

Press the manual mode on the instant cup and set it to 45 minutes.

Perform a quick release after the instant boat countdown.

Add more salt and seasonings if you want.

Add the cabbage and simmer for 5-10 minutes.

Serve and enjoy!

Remarks

This has 6 servings and 2 net carbs per serving.

Sear the meat in batches if you have a smaller Instant Pot.

Always keep the lid of the Instant Pot off when using the cook function.

In manual mode, the Instant Pot takes 10 minutes to pressurize.

Use a wooden spoon to move the vent to the vent position for quick release. Be careful not to burn yourself!

If you want a slightly crunchy cabbage, let it rest for 5 minutes at the end.

nutrition

Calories: 238 kcal | Carbohydrates: 3 g | Protein: 25 g | Fat: 12 g | Saturated fat: 2 g | Cholesterol: 70 mg | Sodium: 181 mg | Potassium: 495 mg | Fiber: 1 g | Sugar: 2 g | Vitamin A: 765 IU | Vitamin C: 35.4 mg | Calcium: 35 mg | Iron: 2.6 mg

23
CHICKEN SOUP WITH COCONUT

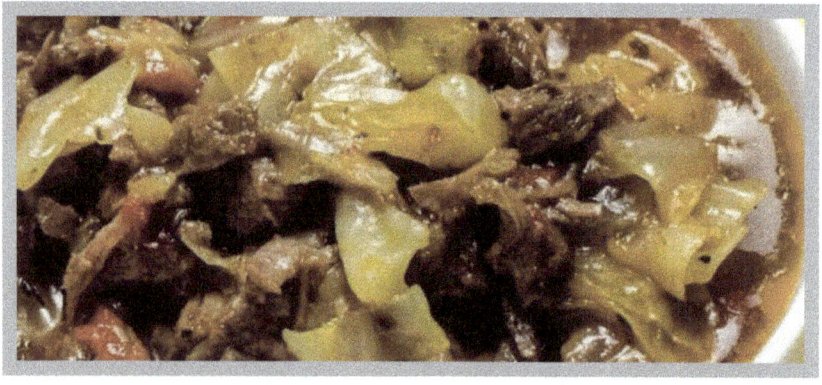

50 MINUTES
Servings: 6

INGREDIENTS
1 pound chicken breast, thinly sliced
Salt and pepper to taste

1 tablespoon. Coconut oil (or vegetable oil)
1 small onion, finely chopped into half moons
2 cloves of garlic, minced
A 1-inch piece of ginger, peeled and finely chopped
1 medium courgette, quartered lengthwise and diced
0.75 pounds of pumpkin, cut into ½-inch cubes (1 cup)
1 red pepper, seeded and thinly sliced
1 small chilli or jalapeño, seeded and thinly sliced
14 oz. light coconut milk (1 can)
2 cups of chicken broth
Juice of 1 lime
A handful of coriander leaves (optional)

PREPARATION

Generously season the chopped chicken breast with salt and pepper.

start by Heating coconut oil in a big pot (5-6 liters) over high heat and add the chicken fillet. Fry over high heat for 4-5 minutes or until the chicken is no longer pink on the outside.

Add the slicedonions, minced garlic and minced ginger. Fry for another 2-3 minutes while stirring.

Add the diced courgettes and diced squash and mix.

Add the sliced pepper, sliced chili or jalapeño pepper, coconut milk, chicken broth, and lime juice. Mix everything well again.

put to a boil, reduce heat, cover and simmer for about 20 minutes or until squash is tender.

Remove from the heat and season with more salt and pepper, if desired. Garnish with cilantro leaves for serving.

. . .

Nutrition Info Per Serving

Nutrition Facts

Coconut Chicken Soup

Amount Per Serving

Calories 231 Calories from Fat 114

% Daily Value*

Fat 12.7g 20%

Saturated Fat 5.5g 28%

Polyunsaturated Fat 0.2g

Monounsaturated Fat 0.2g

Cholesterol 3.7mg 1%

Sodium 45.1mg 2%

Potassium 357.5mg 10%

Carbohydrates 11.6g 4%

Fiber 1.7g 7%

Sugar 5g 6%

Protein 17.1g 34%

Vitamin A 6195IU 124%

Vitamin C 65.2mg 79%

Calcium 19mg 2%

Iron 0.9mg 5%

Net carbs 9.9g

* Percent Daily Values are based on a 2000 calorie diet.

24

INSTANT POT BACON MUSHROOM CAULIFLOWER SOUP

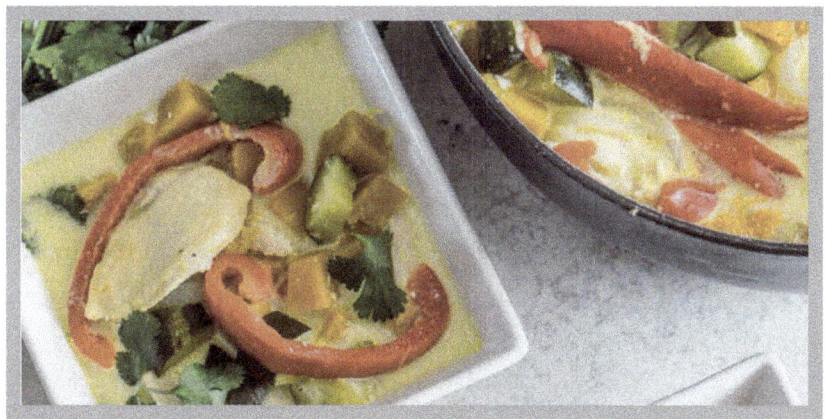

30 MINUTES

Servings: 6

INGREDIENTS

6 slices of bacon, chopped

4 cups of cauliflower florets
4 cups of water or chicken broth for added flavor
8 ounces quartered mushrooms
1/2 cup onion finely chopped
3 cloves of chopped garlic
½ cup of heavy cream
¼ teaspoon chopped red pepper
1 teaspoon of salt

PREPARATION

Fry the bacon and cook until crispy * (this takes about 5 minutes). Scoop the bacon and leave the fat in the instant pot.

Fry the onions for 2-3 minutes, then add the mushrooms and cook for another 2-3 minutes, add the garlic, salt and chilli and stir for another 30 seconds.

Add the water and cauliflower, close the lid, and make sure the stop valve is closed.

Cook in soup mode for 6 minutes (15 minutes to build up and relieve pressure).

Quickly release the pressure after the cook cycle is complete. Add the cream.

Serve the soup and garnish with the crispy bacon.

grades

Note: The nutritional information reflects the use of water as a liquid. If use chicken or vegetable broth, the nutritional values will change.

When adding broth instead of water, add just half a teaspoon of salt and add more at the end if you think you need more.

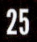

ROAST BEEF SOUP

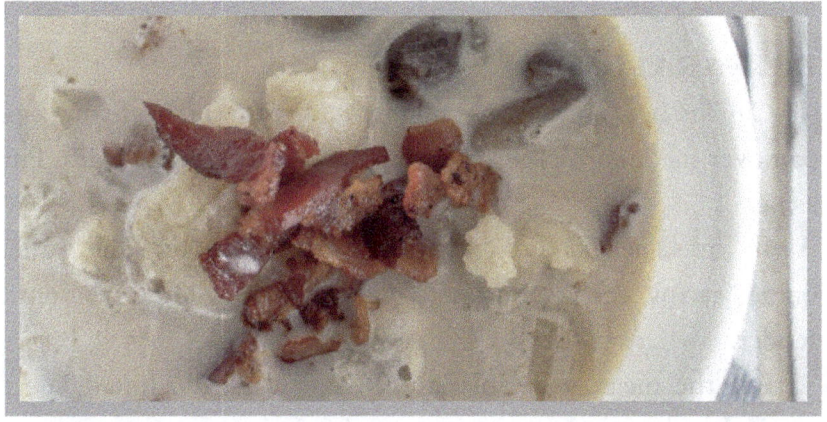

40 MINUTES

Servings 8

INGREDIENTS

1 pound of steamed meat

2 tablespoons of oil
8 cups low-sodium beef broth
1 cup carrots, chopped
2 finely chopped garlic cloves
1 cup celery cubes
1 cup chopped onions
1 cup beetroot, peeled and diced
1 cup diced tomatoes
2 cups of sliced mushrooms
1 teaspoon of dried thyme
1 bay leaf
1 teaspoon of salt
1/4 teaspoon ground pepper

PREPARATION

Cut the beef stew into small pieces. Brown the beef stew in a pan over medium-high heat until golden brown on all sides. Put aside.

In the same pan and add 1 teaspoon of oil, sauté the garlic, onion, carrot, celery and beets. Cook for 3-4 minutes or until tender.

Put the meat, vegetables, diced tomatoes and liquid, meat stock, bay leaf and 1 teaspoon of dried thyme in a saucepan. Cover and then allow i simmer for 20-30 minutes or till the meat is tender.

Remove the lid and add the sliced mushrooms. Cook for another 3-4 minutes until the mushrooms are tender.

Season to taste with salt and pepper, remove the bay leaf and serve!

26
KETO ZUCCHINI BASIL SOUP

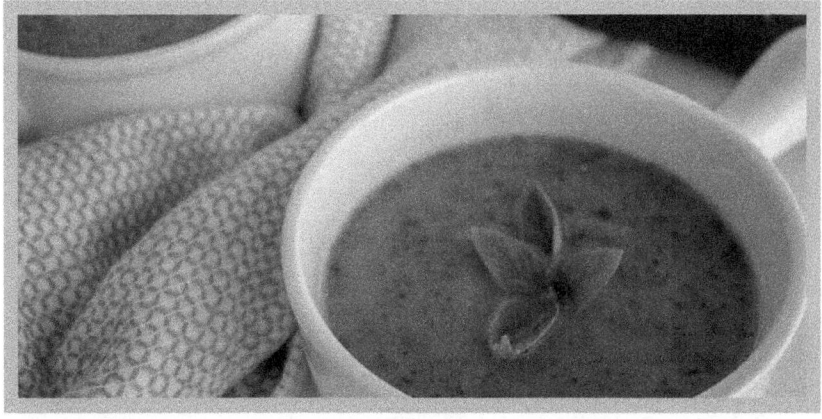

28 min
Servings 4

INGREDIENTS
2 medium zucchini

1 onion, peeled and chopped
2 cloves of garlic, scrape and slice
3 tps of coconut oil or olive oil for coconut without
3 cups of vegetable broth
⅓ cup of fresh basil
½ teaspoon of salt
½ teaspoon white or black pepper

PREPARATION

Heat the oil in a large saucepan.

Add onion and garlic and cook over medium heat for 3-5 minutes until soft.

Slice the zucchini and add to the saucepan. Cook for another 5 minutes, stirring occasionally.

Add the vegetable broth, bring to a boil, cover with a lid and simmer for 15 minutes.

Add the basil and blend with a hand mixer or food processor.

Season to taste and serve

NUTRITION

Serving size: 1 serving
Calories: 87 kcal
Carbohydrates: 6 g
Protein: 2 g
Fat: 7 g
Fiber: 2 g

27

CHEESE SOUP WITH INSTANT LOW-CARBOHYDRATE CHICKEN SAUCE

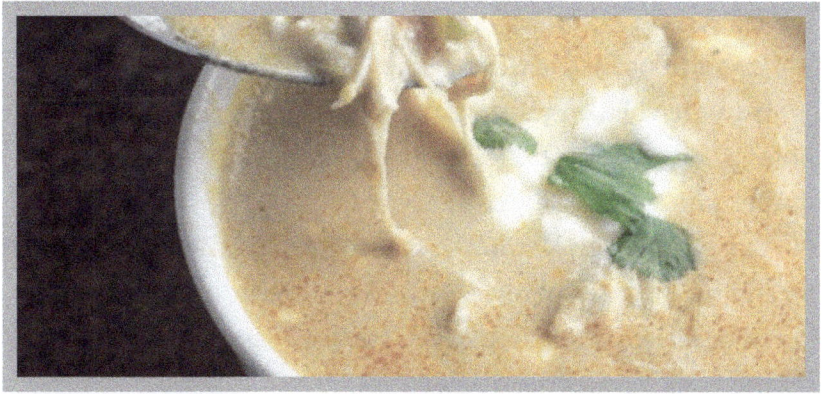

35 min
Servings 6

INGREDIENTS

1 pound boneless and skinless chicken thighs
1 ⅓ cups of red sauce

3 cups of chicken broth

½ teaspoon sea salt

1 teaspoon of garlic powder

½ teaspoon of ground chipotle powder

½ teaspoon of ground black pepper

½ teaspoon ground coriander

½ teaspoon of ground cumin

½ teaspoon dried parsley

1 8-ounce packet of cream cheese, soft and diced

½ cup of jack cheese

¼ cup of crumbled cream cheese

2 tablespoons of chopped coriander optional

PREPARATION

Instant Pot Instructions:

Add the chicken broth, salsa, sea salt, garlic powder, chipotle powder, black pepper, coriander, cumin and parsley to the instant pot.

Put the chicken legs in the saucepan. Cover and also lock the lid and turn the steam release handle to the closed position.

Under High Pressure, select Pressure Cooker (Manual) and set the cooking timer to 20 minutes.

When the cooking time is up, release the pressure naturally for 10 minutes, then quickly release the strain that still exists

With a slotted spoon, remove the chicken thighs from the pot and place them on a cutting board. Create minced chicken with two forks. Put the shredded chicken back in the saucepan and toss it in the soup.

Choose sauté in the Instant Pot and bring the soup to a boil. Put the cream cheese cubes in the saucepan and stir continuously until the cream cheese has dissolved in the soup (good if there are small pieces of unmelted cream cheese).

Press Cancel to turn off the saucepan, add the jack cheese, and stir until it has melted in the soup.

12 tablespoon crumbled queso fresco and 1 teaspoon chopped coriander should be sprinkled on top of each cup of soup. Warm it up and serve.

Instructions for the slow cooker

Put all ingredients except queso fresco and coriander in a 6 liter slow cooker. Cover and simmer for 6-8 hours.

When the slow cooking time is over, just put the chicken on a cutting board and chop it with two forks. Toss the shredded chicken back into the soup in the slow cooker.

Serve the soup in bowls with queso fresco and optional coriander on top. Serve immediately.

28

INSTANT POT CREAMY KETO TACO SOUP

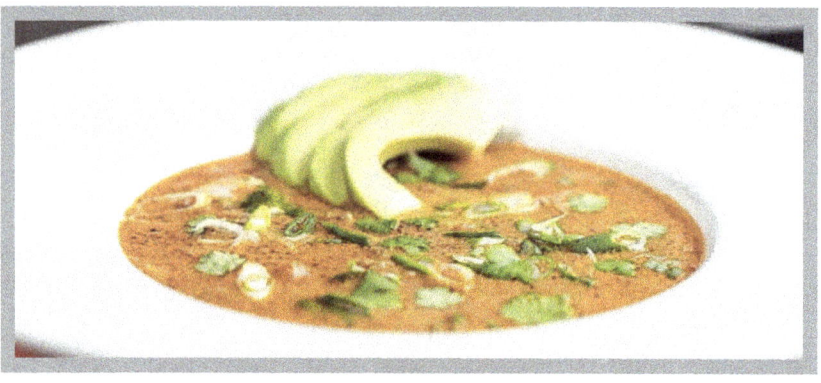

30-MINUTE

Servings 4

INGREDIENTS

1 pound ground beef

1/2 cup onion

1 tablespoon of chopped garlic
1.5 tablespoons of taco seasoning
1 teaspoon of kosher salt
1 cup of water, divided
14 ounces diced tomatoes, 1 can break up
4 ounce whipped cream
1 cup of hot cheddar cheese
1 avocado, sliced (optional)
1/2 cup spring onions, chopped (optional)
1/2 cup cilantro chopped
Optional non-ketogenic ingredients
Beans, cooked
Corn, cooked
Black beans, cooked

PREPARATION

Turn the Instant Pot into a pan. When the indicator is hot, add the ground beef, onion, and garlic. Break open the meat as much as possible. When the meat is no longer in a large lump, add the taco dressing and salt and cook for about 1 minute.

Add ¼ cup of water and mix the Instant Pot Coating thoroughly.

Add the undrained tomatoes and the remaining cup of water.

Close the pot with the lid. Put the Instant Pot on high pressure for 5 minutes. When the cooking time is up, naturally release the pressure on the pan for 10 minutes, then release any remaining pressure.

Open the saucepan and add the whipped cream and cheese. Add more water if needed.

Divide into four bowls and garnish with avocado slices and spring onions, if used, just before serving.

Slow cooker instructions

To make this simple taco soup in your slow cooker, just brown the meat, add the browned meat and all of the ingredients except cheese and heavy whipped cream, and cook on high for 3 hours. Then mix the whipped cream and grated cheese, garnish with avocado slices and spring onions (if used) and serve. Calm.

29

CREAMY LEMON CHICKEN SOUP WITH SPINACH

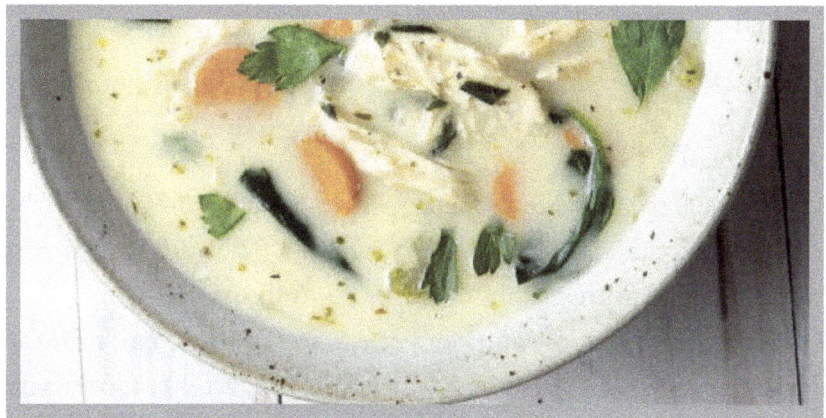

35 MINUTES
Servings: 8

INGREDIENTS

2 tablespoons of butter or olive oil

1 large sweet onion, peeled and minced

1 cup of chopped celery

1 cup carrots, chopped

5-6 garlic cloves, minced

1 pound boneless chicken breast

2 teaspoons lemon zest

1 tablespoon Italian dressing

8 cups of chicken broth

1/2 cup of cream

1/4 cup cornstarch (2 teaspoons glucommanan powder per keto)

1 cup of grated Parmesan cheese

1 cup baby spinach, packed

1/4 cup of chopped parsley

salt and pepper

PREPARATION

Put a large 6-8 liter saucepan over medium heat. Add the butter, onion, and celery. Fry for 3 minutes. Then add the carrots and garlic and sauté for another 2 minutes to soften them.

Add the whole raw chicken breasts to the saucepan. Add the lemon zest, Italian seasoning, chicken broth, 1 teaspoon of salt, and 1/4 teaspoon of black pepper. Cover and bring to boil. try Reduce the heat to low and cook the chicken for about 15 minutes, covered, if necessary.

In a separate cup, whisk together the cream and cornstarch (or glucomannan) until smooth.

Once the chicken is cooked, use the tongs to remove the chicken breast from the pot and place it on a cutting board.

Mix the cream and Parmesan into the base of the soup to

thicken it. Stir for another minute until the Parmesan melts and mixes perfectly with the soup base.

Use two forks to chop the chicken breast. Then mix the shredded chicken, spinach, and parsley into the soup. Taste it, then season with salt and pepper as needed. Serve hot, with the addition of Parmesan if desired!

www.ingramcontent.com/pod-product-compliance
Lightning Source LLC
Chambersburg PA
CBHW071122030426
42336CB00013BA/2168